Hair Raiser

A comprehensive guide for optimizing

hair re growth and hair maintenance

Preface

Before I begin to take you through this journey of hair loss, hair re growth and hair maintenance, I want to tell you why I am uniquely qualified to write this book. Being a member of the less fairer sex, my knowledge is mainly focused on male hair loss and hair re growth, but some of this knowledge will also help female facing hair loss as well. I must stress that I am not a medical professional, I am a layman (albeit a rather intelligent and extremely curious one) - I am just like you, a regular guy who has struggled with hair loss and has been exceptionally persistent in understanding all about it to combat this peculiar human ailment. This book is a culmination of over one and a half decade of research, trial and error, experimentation and dedication to two causes - optimize hair regrowth and hair maintenance. I have read countless academic journals, clinical trial results, studies, blogs, ancient eastern scriptures and texts, videos by doctors, vlogs by youtubers sharing their experiences and advise by nutritionists/physicians. I have also personally tried and tested many methods and combinations of treatments to understand and learn what works best, after dealing with Androgenic Alopecia or male pattern baldness (both at the top and crown of my scalp) since my teenage and after suffering from a very severe, aggressive and wide spreading Alopecia Areata (I had two thirds of my hair fall out at the peak of the disease) when I went through an exceptionally difficult, stressful period in my life. I have successfully treated both of these ailments with each requiring slightly different applications of strategies and methods. After 15 years, I can safely say that I now know exactly what causes hair fall in men, how to eliminate hair fall (or at least slow it down) and promote hair re growth.

Hair re growth depends on many (many!) factors and variables. All the research I have seen so far on hair re growth are quite sporadic. I have not seen all the knowledge relating to hair regrowth aggregated in one place. The main purpose of this book is to bring all of that knowledge together, in one place, so that you do not have to spend a decade and a half (like me) to understand what is involved in preserving, maintaining or re growing your hair. Through this book, I want to help you defeat hair loss and re grow your hair safely without any adverse side effects. This book will summarize all the major factors that contribute to hair fall. I have deliberately not gone into the detailed literature of this very complex area of medical science, as doing that would defeat the purpose of this book, which is to simply and succinctly communicate in one place what causes hair fall, how you can eliminate it and how you can promote hair re growth. And, this book will sprout into a 10,000 page monstrosity! I have referenced the detailed science wherever possible, if you are interested in looking more deeply into the topics I will discuss. Another point to note is that all the sections of this book is inter-connected, so to fully appreciate and understand all the complex processes involved in eliminating hair loss, kick-starting hair re growth and maintain your hair at the most optimal level, I would strongly recommend that you read the entire book and not skip any of the sections.

Debunking Myths

There are no magic pills, potions, serums or a single product that will combat hair loss. I have seen numerous "experts" claim that they have developed a single product that tackles hair fall and/or re grow hair, but I can explicitly tell you that this is simply not possible. There are too many variables involved in the biology of hair for any single product to tackle all in one go. Additionally, as you read on, you will see that there are internal and external factors involved in maintaining the optimum health of your hair, so just one pill (intended for internal use) or just one serum (intended for external use) physically will not be able to tackle both aspects.

I have seen countless people claim that they have found a miracle cure for their hair fall. In a lot of these cases, it is vital not to confuse correlation (which could be only one factor) with causation (which is likely to be numerous factors which are likely to be interdependent). For example, I have seen some people swear by onion juice that has completely reversed their hair loss. Yes, onion juice can have some positive effects on the health of your scalp and hair follicles by acting as an anti-inflammatory agent, which might reduce hair fall. However, it will certainly not reverse hair fall completely, neither will it enhance the health of hair to its optimum level. Someone can observe reversal of, say Alopecia Areata related hair loss (more details on this form of hair loss later), after using onion juice in affected bald patches, but the reversal might have occurred due to changes in other lifestyle factors, general reduction in stress and additional reduction in bodily inflammation (not just because of the usage of onion juice). So it follows logic that it cannot be claimed onion juice reversed the Alopecia Areata.

I have also observed that many actual experts in many forums and platforms only speak about one or two legitimate factor that contributes to hair loss and recommends methods on tackling it, without dissecting the ailment from all possible angles. A handy coincidence in such cases is that they are expert in only that one field they discuss. For instance, a nutritionist only tends to focus on the dietary elements that contributes to or reduces hair fall, without expanding on the hair loss topic or a dermatologist only focuses on the external cosmetic scalp treatments that might reduce hair fall without referring to any internal biology that could be affecting a subject. Such tunnel vision is quite dangerous as the subject might follow the treatment or recommendation, see no results and give up after a while as this isolated approach is tackling the core problem that is leading to hair fall. Diet and health of the scalp's skin might be valid factors contributing only partly to hair loss, but only treating these two factors in isolation might not result in any positive changes. Isolation treatment will only work if a subject has a specific problem related to a specific factor only and nothing else - such as some deficiency in their diet or a scalp skin condition; and assuming (this a very big assumption here) all the other factors that contribute to hair loss does are functioning at peak capacity. These isolated views of hair loss are given further legitimacy by these professionals through confirmation bias. You will find that these experts will only refer to a study or a clinical trial that confirms their findings or hypothesis. They will not refer to any other unrelated findings that detail some other reason for hair loss or any contradictory finding that will have a negative impact on the view they are presenting. For example, a dermatologist who is promoting, say, a shampoo with a certain active ingredient, might only refer to studies that show why that ingredient stimulates the scalp and hair re growth (without ever referring to hormonal studies for instance that provides a different view for hair loss) or a study that show such shampoos having little or no negligible effect on hair loss.

There is no silver bullet that will stop your hair loss and there is no instant gratification. Not just one thing will yield the optimum result, it will need to be a culmination of many and varied efforts that will need to come together to gain the best results. Anyone who tells you otherwise is a snake oil salesman. It is a long, attritional process, which will demand your dedication and test your patience. Male pattern baldness or Androgenic Alopecia will need regular attention for the entirety of your life. You cannot expect to treat it for a few months and leave it. Left unchecked, Androgenic Alopecia will rear its ugly hear (quite literally!). Alopecia Areata or sudden patchy baldness will need regular attention and treatment until it is completely eliminated. However, after eliminating it, you will still need to be mindful of its trigger so that you do not allow it to develop again in the future. You will also need to invest a lot of time, effort and money. However, it is all worth it - you are putting everything in to develop your hair and your general health. As you read on, you will appreciate all the positive health benefits that you

are able to realize if you embark on this journey of improving the
health of your hair.

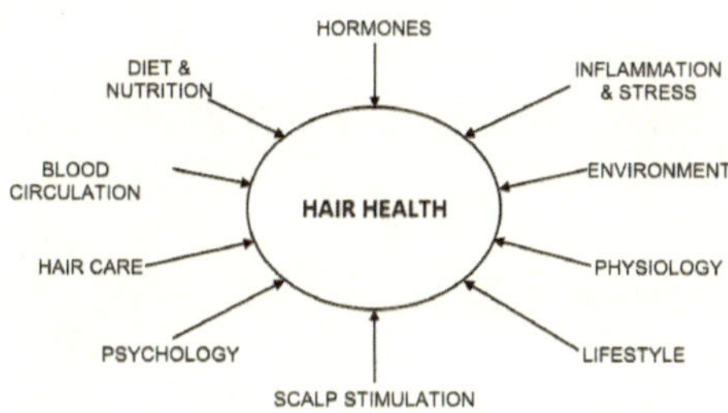

Different Factors Affecting Hair Loss

The unique perspective of this book is that it tackles the hair
loss problem comprehensively from every single angle and treats it
as almost a mathematical problem which has a definite solution.
This book is all about maximizing reduction of hair loss, maximizing hair re growth and maximizing the good health of hair through
maintenance by using a combination of methods and techniques,
both internal and external, to achieve absolute optimal, peak results.
This views or recommendations set out in this book are not 'philoso-
phies' or opinions, they are all deduced from hard, scientific facts
and all conclusions made are evidence based. The hair loss problem
is tackled from every angle, with no stones unturned and every
linkage/inter-dependencies are explored, which is distinct in this
not very well understood discipline of human biology. This book
does not make any outlandish claims or assertions that you may find
in other places. The only goal of this book is to find the maximizing
point of optimal hair health for individuals. This optimal point will

Hormones

Several hormones contribute to hair fall and hair re growth.

Dihydrotestosterone (DHT)

Hormones are arguably the most important factor that leads to hair loss. The most widely quoted nemesis of male hair follicles is DHT. DHT production is associated with hair follicle shrinkage and eventual termination of hair growth. DHT production will lead to male pattern baldness in those who are genetically susceptible to hair loss. A key thing to note is that, unlike what many would have you believe, DHT is not a "bad" hormone. In fact, it is a vital hormone that human (and especially men) produce naturally. It is inextricably linked with body growth and self-regulation, metabolic activities and development of sexual characteristics.

There are many ways to block DHT to promote hair re growth. A very popular method is to ingest prescription medication such as Finasteride, which contains a formula to inhibit 5 alpha reductase that synthesizes DHT from testosterone in areas like the prostrate, hair follicles, testes and adrenal glands. Another method (often paired with prescription medication) is the application of Azelaic acid on the scalp to stop the 5 alpha reductase to interact with the scalp.

If you are considering using the two medications above, I would strongly advise you to not proceed. I found both Finasteride and Azelaic acid to have extremely adverse side effects, mainly affecting my sexual health. I have read many accounts of people suffering from the same effects. Some clinical trials (often conducted or financed by the manufacturers of these products) suggest that there are no or very low side effects. Perhaps some people are immune to the potential adverse side effects of these prescription medication or perhaps their genetic make-up enables them to use these medications safely, it is a little bit like using growth hormones to build muscles - some people will get the desired results but for some it can be catastrophic.

As I mentioned above, I recommend sticking to natural remedies (of which there are plenty) to counter the adverse side effects of DHT and retaining its positive effects. I use Saw Palmetto and Stinging Root Nettle tea to counter the side effects of DHT without any adverse side effects. In fact, aside from reducing my hair loss by eliminating the adverse side effects of DHT, my prostrate health has got better (I can sleep through the night without needing to go to the toilet) and my sexual health has come back to normal after a period of near impotence due to the use of prescription medication.

The diagram below lists the different types of male pattern baldness across different maturity levels. Type A is baldness that affects the front of the head, Type O affects the crown, Type M affects the Parietal Ridge or the top corners of the forehead and Type O + M affects both the crown and the Parietal Ridge simultaneously.

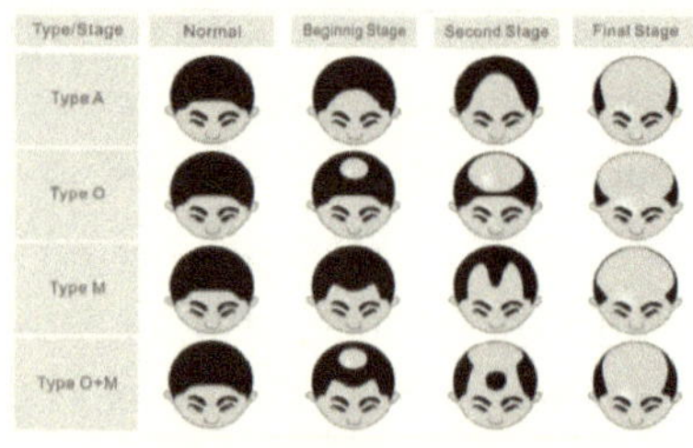

Androgenic Alopecia or Male Pattern Baldness

Cortisol & Stress

The other hormone which can trigger hair fall is cortisol. Cortisol is released by the body through the adrenal glands and is very important in helping the body respond to stress. There is good stress (e.g. stress we feel during exercising) and bad stress (e.g. chronic anxiety or fear). Bad stress can cause damage to the adrenal glands, can cause inflammation in the body and can cause the body to produce Cortisol abnormally. This can wreak havoc in the normal functioning of your immune system and anti-bodies. The manifestation of inflammation in your body can be quite mild (e.g. you might get a few acnes or suffer from a cold for a day or two) or it can be much more serious (e.g. diabetes or arthritis). Your white blood cells might start attacking the body itself during periods of such bad stress, mistaking, for instance, hair follicles as foreign invaders (like the anti-bodies would if a virus were to attack the body). Such behaviour of the body is called auto-immune disease. Very little is known about the exact mechanisms that lead to the trigger of auto-immune diseases. Only 2% of the population is affected by such diseases although it is on the increase, quite possible due to rapid environmental and dietary changes leading to small but noticeable mutation of humans. Auto-immune diseases are associated with a plethora of symptoms, including Alopecia Areata (patchy hair loss mostly at the back or side of the head where hair follicles are attacked by white blood cells), Psoriasis, Celiac disease and so on.

Here, we will focus on Alopecia Areata. I have suffered from this disease for over four years. If you have it, I would suggest that you should investigate the underlying cause - e.g. what is causing you bad stress? Is it your lifestyle or lack of sleep? Are you on a very unhealthy diet? Are you chronically depressed or anxious? You MUST tackle the underlying cause to eliminate Alopecia Areata. While you are tackling the underlying cause, if you are desperate to get your hair back, dermatologists will usually recommend steroids to combat anti-bodies that are attacking your hair follicles. The most commonly prescribed steroid to tackle Alopecia Areata are Corticosteroid injections such as Triamicilone Acetonide to the affected regions of the scalp to counter the inflammation in the area (which would normally be countered, if at all required by your body, by natural Cortisol production with its anti-inflammatory properties) and to push the white blood cells away so that they do not attack the hair follicles. Intra-muscular steroids with Methylprednisolone

Acetate such as Depomedrone might also be prescribed to regulate the immune system and to complement the Corticosteroid treatment. These treatments can have severe side effects - for example, Corticosteroids can damage the bone mass of the skull and long-term use can lead to diabetes, osteoporosis, rapid weight gain or weight loss and weakening of the immune system. Usually after 6 months of steroid treatments, hairs begin to reappear in patches. This treatment is very effective in the short term, but many patients relapse, and their hair falls out in clumps again if the underlying cause of the auto-immune disease is not tackled. Dermatologists usually prescribe ointments containing corticosteroids if the injections do not work, but these ointments are far less effective (although they have far fewer side effects). In a nutshell, if you have severe Alopecia Areata, steroid injections might be necessary but to prevent the and eliminate the disease, the underlying cause (i.e. the cause of the bad stress) must be eliminated. The steroid treatments can be quite costly, depending on what your dermatologist charges for consultation and each session of steroid therapy. The underlying cause might be anything ranging from lifestyle, your psychological state, poor diet or environmental factor. Only you will be able to answer what recent change has triggered this inflammatory response from your body and then you will need to reverse that change to defeat Alopecia Areata. It is natural for about 100 hair follicles to shed daily. If your hair fall is significantly higher than this or if it is falling out in clumps or if you have developed a sudden bald patch in one or more areas of your scalp, your body might well have been through some kind of shock due to psychological or physiological stress or a radical change in diet or the environment. If it is the case, something will need to change. Act immediately to mitigate these adverse effects. Below is a patient suffering from Alopecia Areata.

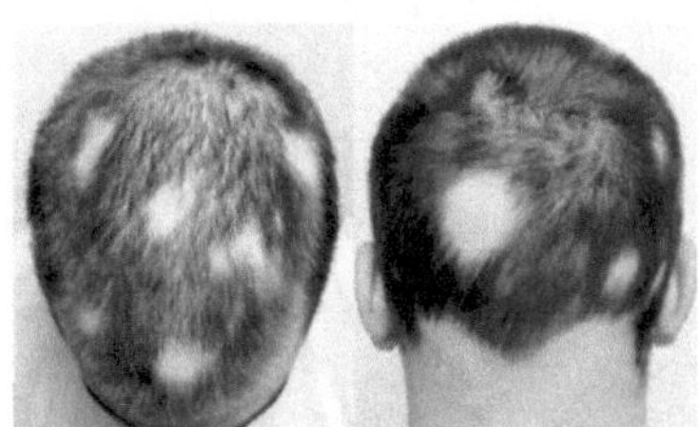

Alopecia Areata or Patchy Hair Loss

There are two other hair fall terminologies that is worth mentioning apart from the two most common ones - Androgenic Alopecia and Alopecia Areata. They are called Alopecia Totalis (a situation where all the hair follicles on the scalp are lost) and Alopecia Universalis (a rare condition where every hair follicle in the body, including eye brows, body hair and facial hair, is lost). In general, the larger the damage, the more difficult it is to reverse the hair fall. If your Alopecia Areata has large patches of bald areas on your scalp, it will be harder to reverse than if you have small patches. It is extremely difficult to reverse Alopecia Totalis, even with steroid treatments. It is almost impossible to reverse Alopecia Unversalis. Luckily, Totalis and Universalis are very rare (at least for now). Androgenic Alopecia (or male pattern, hereditary baldness) is the most common form of hair loss (accounting for 95% of all hair loss) affecting a very large part of matured men (by the age of 35, two-thirds of all men are affected by some form of hair thinning), followed by Alopecia Areata (auto-immune diseases that trigger Alopecia Areata affects about 2% of the population - men and women). Alopecia Totalis and Universalis are much less common but reliable data about these are not readily available. If you have any form of Alopecia that is not Androgenic (or hereditary male pattern baldness), your body is most likely suffering from some form of stress and/or inflammation. So, your strategy to tackle this ailment should be to remove the any stress (be it psychological or physiological) and reduce any inflammation however you can, so that hormones and your bodily functions (such as normal functioning of white blood cell) come back to normal. The main principle to do this is ensure you are doing everything you can (however small) and are tackling the stress/inflammation problem from all angles (be it through diet, environment or lifestyle changes). The reason for this is that there is, as yet, no known method of isolating the cause of this stress/ailment, which if tackled, would alleviate the Alopecia from progressing and kick-start the hair re growth process - therefore, the most prudent approach is to ensure all bases are covered as much as possible. However, bear in mind that even even with a cocktail of steroids, it will take several months to reverse Alopecia Areata. It will take even longer (usually close to a year) to cure Alopecia Areata naturally, but sustainably.

All Other Hormones

Finally, if you can ensure that all of your glands (pituitary, adrenal, thyroid, etc.) are functioning properly and your hormones are naturally produced at the optimum level (neither over nor under produced), are all working in unison and are in-sync with each other

Diet & Nutrition

The saying goes - "You are what you eat". Your hair is no exception, it will be what you feed it and your diet will play an essential role in the health of your hair. Your hormones, no one vitamin, mineral, nutrient or supplement will rectify hair loss or promote hair re growth. You will need to have a diverse and healthy diet to maximize the nutrition to your hair follicles, that is rich in all the necessary vitamins, minerals, essential fats and protein. A key point to note is that, whenever possible, you want to get all these nutrients from clean, organic, natural sources (be it fruits, vegetables, meat or drinks) rather than through refined sugar, deep fried food, processed food or prescription/non-prescription medication. For instance, your body will absorb a lot less vitamin C from a pill compared with an organic Orange. Also, try to have a wide variety of food in your diet. This is because the composition of each food and the way we absorb nutrients from each food is extremely complex and depends on a myriad of factors. A wide diversity of food sources ensures all of your nutrient needs are met and properly absorbed by the body all year round. Additionally, avoid any refined sugar, gluten, unnatural, man-made food with preservatives or food exposed to toxins such as pesticides or harmful fertilizers, especially if you are susceptible to inflammation and you wish to eliminate the risk of triggering auto-immune diseases such as Alopecia Areata.

It is harder to source some nutrients directly from readily available food - when this is the case, I recommend filling these nutrition gap through herbal, natural supplements, ideally in powdered form (or as a capsule if powdered supplement is not available). However, supplements are just what they are named as - they are secondary nutrition source meant to complement your main diet. You cannot rely on supplements alone to support your hair follicles, your primary diet (i.e. the real food you intake as meals throughout the day) is more important than supplements. A rich, healthy, diverse diet with some (varied) supplements will work together to maximize the health benefits and as a positive side effect, you will notice improvement in your hair's health as well.

Vitamins

Going into a more granular level, you should ensure you are not deficient in any vitamins - you should have adequate levels of vitamins A, B, C, D, E, K and all its sub constituent vitamins (e.g. B12 is a sub constituent of Vitamin B). All vitamins will work in unison for your good health and hair (are you starting to see a pattern here?). Some vitamins are more essential (such as Vitamins E, which improves the blood circulation and helps the follicles work more efficiently to promote hair growth and Vitamin A, which is responsible for hair/tissue repair and growth) for hair follicles than others, but all contribute to healthy hair by working together and complementing each other. To ensure you are getting the right vitamins, very simply and without getting into the technical details, as a rule of thumb you should look to eat five colours of fruits and vegetables. There is debate about the proportion of fruit or vegetable you should look to eat when abiding by this five colour principle but in general, if you have 3 portions of fruits and 2 portions of vegetables (or vice versa), of five different colours, it will more than suffice. Try to have seasonal fruits and vegetables with leafy greens such as Spinach or Broccoli as a staple and make sure you do not consume the same fruits and vegetables over and over again. Look to diversify your intake of these colours and have fun with it - try out exotic or rare breeds of fruits and vegetables! This practice will not only help your hair, but it will also boost your health immensely.

Minerals

On the same vein, you should look to ensure you are getting all the essential minerals such as magnesium, iron, zinc, calcium, iodine and so on. Again, some minerals such as magnesium and zinc are more important for the health of your hair than others but if you make sure you are not deficient in any of these, they will all work together for your hair and your overall health. Magnesium, specifically, can be have really effect de-stressing effects and help calm the mind, in addition to providing nutrition for the body and the hair. Magnesium can be sourced from food, taken as a supplement (Biotin supplements, for example, are rich in magnesium) and can be sprayed on which will then be absorbed by the skin and enter the bloodstream. Good quality, organic dairy, meat, grains and beans are full of these essential minerals. Again, like vitamin sources, look to have a diverse variety of mineral sources in your diet. Additionally, if you ensure you are having your five a day, as suggested in the previous paragraph, they will go a long way in meeting all your body's mineral needs. Another unlikely source of good minerals is the humble drinking water, especially if it is (drumbeats!) Mineral Water! Clean, high quality fresh water from streams or mountains are much richer in nutrients than tap water most of us drink (and Mineral Water tastes delicious as well with a sweet, crisp taste) and are not adulterated/recycled with any chemicals such as chlorine, fluoride. Of course, mineral water is expensive, so if at all possible, try to drink mineral water in the morning to give your body an early mineral boost. Since 60% of our body is actually water, it is essential that you are drinking it from a good source and are getting plenty of it.

Proteins, Essential Fats & Biotin

Hair is made almost entirely of protein, specifically a fibrous structural protein called Keratin. So, it goes without saying that proteins are vital for the health of your hair. Most Western diets contain enough protein for the hair. However, again building on the concepts developed above, look to get your protein from organic and diverse sources. Free range, organic eggs are an excellent source of protein. High quality red and white meat are also great for feeding your hair follicles. Controversially, soy protein (from organic tofu for example) can help in the development of hair, but for men, studies have shown that soy protein can increase Estrogen levels which might not be desirable for overall male health as Estrogen has been linked to reduction in Testosterone, libido and weight gain in men. Omega 3 fatty acids nourish the hair and support thickening. Nuts, seeds and fresh water fish are great sources of such fats - almonds, walnuts, Flaxseeds, Pumpkin seeds and Salmon Trout are all great sources of this (but again, remember the diversification rule). Other fats such as monounsaturates from natural sources such as Avocado are great at maintaining the natural oil and PH level balance of the scalp, which if unbalanced can lead to clogging of hair follicles and stop hair growth. However, avoid trans-fat which are usually found in processed food such as cookies, donuts and deep-fried food. Whole grains such as Sourdough bread are rich in biotin along with iron, zinc and B vitamins. Biotin is required for cell proliferation and plays an important part in producing amino acids (protein) which are required for your hair to grow.

Supplements, Probiotics & Fermented Food

Aside from maintaining a well-rounded diet, some diet supplementation (from organic, natural sources) can improve the health of your hair even further. When I say "supplement", I do not mean anything unnatural, man-made or prescription-based medication. Supplements simply mean food which are not necessarily abundant in a healthy diet or are difficult to source from everyday food. As I mentioned in chapter 2, Saw Palmetto and Root Nettle combat DHT and directly contribute to reducing hair fall resulting from the harmful compounds produced by DHT (i.e. 5 Alpha reductase). Asides from the beneficial effect on your hair, these supplements improve the health of your facial hair and prostrate as well.

Some supplements help in detoxification of the liver, improve blood circulation throughout the body (including circulation to the scalp), help combat inflammation and are rich in anti-oxidants, which all have beneficial effects for the health of your hair. These include Ashwagandha, Ginseng, Moringa, Wheatgrass and Green Tea. Additionally, Mucuna Pruriens (supplement for improving thyroid health) and L-Dopa (supplement for helping build essential amino acids and improving health of glands), also improve health of hair and your general health.

If you feel you are not getting enough essential vitamins or minerals from your diet, you might want to use supplements to cover these shortfalls. However, as discussed above, natural sources of vitamins and minerals are more effective as they are absorbed better by our bodies. If you do need supplementation for vitamins and minerals, make sure you are using a high quality, well reviewed manufacturer. Look out for the essential hair vitamins (A, C, D and E), Iron, Zinc and specifically vitamin B complex (also known as Biotin). Biotin improves health of hair follicles, skin and nails, so it is essential that your diet provides you sufficient levels of natural Biotin, but if it does not, then the shortfall should be covered with supplements.

Bone broth is a fantastic source of essential fats, proteins, minerals, calcium and collagen, which is not common in a Western diet. Bone broth has positive effects on supporting the normal functioning of the immune system, boosts detoxification, aids metabolism and promotes anabolism. All of this helps improve the health of your hair, as well as your joints, skin and gut health.

You might be surprised to know that some studies have linked the health of the gut to Alopecia Areata. If your gut is not absorbing nutrients from food properly and is not releasing these nutrients into your bloodstream, toxins can start accumulating in your body and can lead to the development of auto-immune diseases, a form of manifestation of which can be Alopecia Areata. The health of the gut is directly correlated with the diverse types of bacteria it hosts. If the bacterial diversity (or bacteria count) is low in the gut, it can trigger the onset of auto-immune diseases and inflammation. Therefore, it is essential that your diet is rich in fermented food and probiotics such as yogurt, pickle, Kimchi, Kombucha or fermented milk.

Finally, to conclude the chapter on diet, intermittent fasting can help detoxify the body and reduce inflammation. When the body is given a break from breaking down calories, it cleanses itself and releases toxins built up over time. There is good evidence to suggest that a longer two to three day fast is more effective in cleansing the body than a shorter fast, especially for obese people (who are more likely to have toxin build up) and for people who have not done intermittent fasting before. Generally, at least 16 hours of intermittent fasting two to three times a week has great cleansing effects on the body in addition to boosting metabolism, supporting weight loss, tissue recovery and whole host of other health benefits.

Some key supplements for hair health and hair re growth are below.

Hair Care

So far, the discussion has been focused on the internal aspects of the biology that impact the health of hair. However, external dermatological and cosmetic aspects, specifically hair and scalp care, can also play a crucial role in reducing hair fall, stimulate hair re growth and help maintain optimum health of hair. Again, it is worth emphasizing that an optimal hair maintenance regimen involves the usage of a diverse range of hair products and techniques. As touched upon earlier, it is essential to ensure that the head and scalp is receiving adequate blood circulation and nutrients both internally and externally. It is also essential that blood circulation to the head/scalp is aided through various mechanisms and that the scalp is receiving a diverse range of nutrients. Previous chapters have already discussed the essential hair nutrients that should be consumed so that internal bodily functions are optimized. So only external nutrients will be discussed in this chapter. In general, whenever you consider using a hair product or think about a hair care routine, always think about blood circulation and nutrients the product or routine will provide.

Blood Circulation & Scalp Stimulation

There are many techniques that can help improve blood circulation to the head and the scalp. If all the internal bodily functions are working properly, it will go a long way in ensuring good blood circulation to the head and distribution of essential nutrients through the bloodstream. However, this internal process can be further optimized and supported through external methods as well. A good (but very painful) way to stimulate the scalp is through dermarolling. Dermarolling is the process of creating micro punctures in the epidermis layer of the skin, usually done to increase collagen production (collagen helps skin tissue repair and fresh skin cell re growth), which gives the skin elasticity, softens scars/wrinkles and can combat acne, by stimulating the affected region of the skin. Dermarolling on the scalp (or anywhere else on the body's skin) achieves similar effects. It is not necessary or advisable to bleed the surface of the scalp, more/strong or frequent dermarolling is not necessarily better; it may, in some cases, only serve to reduce the good effects of dermarolling. Only ensure the scalp turns pink or reddish and stop the dermarolling process - when you get to this stage, you can see blood rushing into the scalp changing the colour of the scalp, which is sufficient. Dermarolling once a month can be very effective in stimulating hair re growth, improve blood circulation to the scalp and help the scalp better absorb nutrients from cosmetic application of hair products. For example, applying oil on the scalp after a dermarolling session can be more effective than only applying oil without any dermarolling, as the scalp is more likely to absorb the oil into the scalp after being stimulated through dermarolling.

Yoga techniques such as head stands are another method of externally inducing blood circulation to the head, which could be done once a week. Deep, mindful breathing and meditation can also improve blood and oxygen circulation throughout the body, including

the head, which will further reinforce the positive effects of stimulating the scalp along with the techniques described above. Regular car-
dio vascular exercises and resistance training (i.e. weight lifting)
with diverse range of movements can also have positive effects on
improving blood circulation throughout the body and up to the
head.

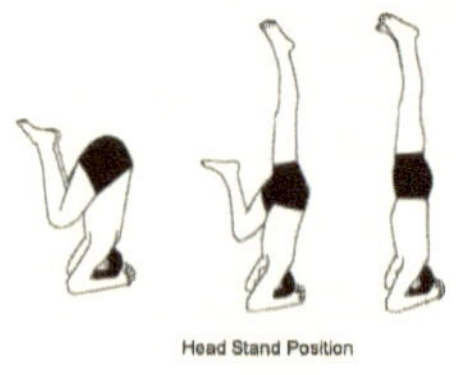

Hair Products

When choosing hair products, keeping with the theme of the
rest of this book, I strongly recommend natural, organic, clean ingredients to obtain key nutrients externally through the scalp. One of
the best sources of feeding the scalp with good nutrients is through
application of oil. Nutrients present in hair and scalp oils are extremely important for maintaining the health of your hair. Again, diversity of oil is important. Look to use many differently kinds of oil
on the scalp by rigorously massaging them into the scalp. Each will
have properties others will not, each will provide a key nutrient in
an amount that cannot be obtained from a different oil and each oil
will complement the other. Organic mustard oil's spice and heat is
great for scalp stimulation. Natural crushed red chilli seed powder
can be added to mustard oil to achieve a more pronounced stimula-

tion effect on the scalp - the scalp will literally burn or itch initially, depending on the amount of chillis used, as blood rushes to the scalp. Black seed oil has anti-histamines and anti-inflammatory properties. Castor oil has anti-bacterial properties, is a great source of omega 3 fatty acids and vitamin E. Coconut and extra virgin olive oil is good for nourishing and moisturizing the scalp. Jojoba oil is rich in iodine which helps combat fungal diseases like dandruff and reduces dryness of the scalp. Other essential oils rich in the nutrients include - Cedarwood, Clary Sage, Aragon, Lavender, Peppermint, Rosemary and Ylang Ylang. The key here is to have variety. A cocktail of all these oils in one serum can work just as well as using these oils in rotation. Application of hair oil once a week or twice a month, ideally via deep head massages for five to ten minutes to aid absorption of nutrients and stimulation, is sufficient. Some parallels to facial skin care can be drawn here. If you have oily skin, you will need less moisturizer but if you have dry, flaky skin, you will need more moisturizer. Or, if you have a skin condition, it will need treatment through application of an ointment. Similarly, if your scalp is dry or has a nutrient deficiency, it will require more frequent oil treatment.

Another great source of scalp nutrient is heena (or Lawsonia Inermis). Heena application can be messy and time consuming but it has very strong anti-inflammatory properties and has nutrients that strengthens, nourishes and moisturizes the hair naturally. Heena does not alter dark hair colours but can slightly alter lighter hair colours, which may or may not be desirable. Heena is also a very effective, natural conditioner for the hair.

To enhance the effects of oil and/or heena on the scalp and to enrich the nutrient content applied to the scalp, Onion and Garlic juice can be blended to create a mixture for your hair. Both Onion and Garlic are nutrient dense root vegetables with great anti-inflammatory properties, which will enhance the health of your scalp. Liquid inside Vitamin E capsules can also be cut out and added to oil or heena mixtures for further enrichment. However, it is not advisable to mix oil with heena as oils do not allow heena absorption into the scalp. Finally, it cannot be emphasized enough that it is necessary to thoroughly massage the oils, heena or mixtures into the scalp to give nutrients the best chance of getting absorbed. Dermarolling before application of these nutrients is even better, as stated above, coupled with thorough massaging of the scalp. This will maximize the blood flow to the scalp and optimize the nutrient absorption. During this process, it is natural for a lot of hair fall to occur; be rest assured that this is normal. Humans shed as much as 100 follicles of hair each day. Also, whatever hair falls out during this process are dead hair follicles that would fall out anyways, so do not be disheartened or worry about this at all. Again, as stated previously, application of oil twice a month is usually sufficient (but dermaroll only once a month).

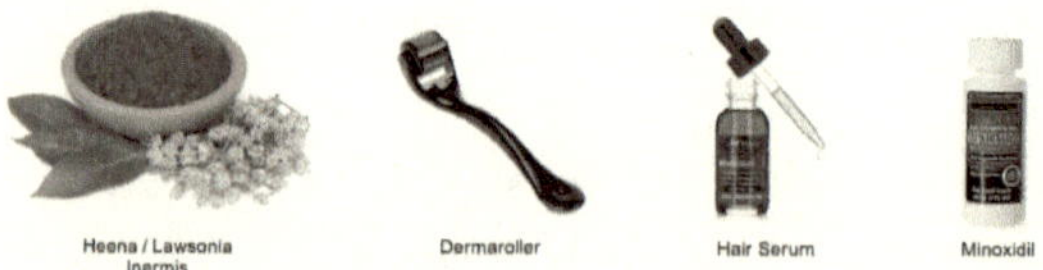

I would very strongly recommend avoiding any hair artificial hair colours (most permanent hair dye contain Paraphenylenediamine or PPD and ammonia) which can damage the proteins in the hair and weaken the hair follicles. I would also discourage usage of any artificial hair products such as hair gels, sprays or any other stylers, as almost all of them contain undesirable artificial substances which are harmful to the health of hair, difficult to get rid of without shampooing frequently and can lead to breakage of hair.

Contemporary caffeine shampoos are quite good for stimulating blood circulation in the scalp. Some even contain natural ingredients that block the harmful compounds of DHT hormone to help prevent hair loss. I recommend shampooing no more than twice a week. Shampooing too frequently can cause the moist hair to break during shower and during drying. Additionally, the scalp does not benefit from shampooing more than a couple of times a week anyways. It is a bit like consuming excess vitamins in one meal - the body just will not absorb it; the body will only absorb the necessary amount and excrete out the excess. Caffeine shampoos, like oil, should be thoroughly massaged into the scalp to aid absorption and should be kept unperturbed for ten minutes, before rinsing off with luke warm water (very hot water can weaken hair follicles). Conditioners can be used once or twice a month, but if oils are used fastidiously and frequently, it can be superfluous.

After shower, to prevent breakage, it is best to gently towel dry the hair ensuring sure as little water residue is left in the hair as possible. Blow drying, especially at high temperature can lead to vulnerable, thin, weak hair follicles to break more easily than towel drying, so it is best avoided. On towel dried hair, a non-greasy serum should be used to combat frizz, tangles and breakage. Hair should generally be combed twice a day, which will ensure adequate blood circulation to the scalp daily, will clear any tangles and keep the hair tidy and clean. Any unnecessary handling of the hair should be avoided. The hair should be brushed (which is very different from combing) once every two or three days - brushing is usually more rigorous than combing, will achieve a better cleaning effect and stimulate blood circulation to the scalp. However, brushing too frequently can damage hair follicles and cause breakage, as its strength is much higher than combing. Therefore, it is best to be prudent with brushing the hair whilst combining it with more regular combing.

The only non-natural (but safe) hair product that I endorse is the application of Minoxidil 5% on the scalp two or three times a week, without any other chemicals such as Azelaic Acid added on to the Minoxidil. Minoxidil in liquid form works best and the 5% formula has the optimum potency. Minoxidil 2% is too weak whereas anything above Minoxidil 5% is excess that is not absorbed by the scalp. Minoxidil can be purchased in non-liquid forms such as foams, but again, the liquid form is the most potent and most effective in combatting hair loss. The best time for application of Minoxidil on the scalp through thorough massage (like application of oil) is 30 minutes to 1 hour before going to sleep. Some people have noted negative side effects of Minoxidil, but closer examination will reveal that 12% Minoxidil with Azelaic Acid is the main culprit, leading to negative consequences such as loss of libido. The standard 5% Minoxidil does have some minor side effects - it can cause dry or itchy scalp as it may contain alcohol which helps scalp absorption and it can cause mild headache. However, it does not have any long term or recurring negative side effects. Building on the same principle of nutrient absorption above, dermarolling, coupled with thorough massage, will lead to best results.

I recommend getting a haircut every month, if hair is growing at a normal rate of one to two inches per month. It is usually best to keep the hair relatively short, ensuring tips are managed so that there are no split ends and so that hair strands do not become too heavy for the hair follicles (or hair roots) to support. There is no concrete evidence that suggests shaving off hair improves strength of hair follicles or stimulates new hair re growth. Shaving the head might make it easier to apply hair products on the scalp but the effect would be negligible overall.

So, packing all of the above in daily, weekly, bi-weekly and monthly frequencies, a good routine could look like:

Daily: comb twice a day; no unnecessary handling of hair; no daily shampooing

Weekly: apply Minoxidil 5% two to three times a week before going to bed; brush hair before taking shower; wash your hair twice a week using a high-quality Caffeine shampoo followed by gentle but thorough towel drying and anti-frizz potion application to avoid breakage; meditate and focus on breathing two to three times a

Lifestyle

Lifestyle can play a major part in the health of your hair. If you are suffering from stress or inflammation due to psychological, physiological and/or environmental reasons, the health of your hair will be affected. So, it is absolutely vital that you have a healthy, positive lifestyle that does not over expose you to stress or causes inflammation to your body. Some degree of stress in this modern day and age is unavoidable but it is essential that you are able to manage the levels of stress and whenever possible, look to detoxify yourself physically to reduce toxin build-up and to reduce inflammation.

Psychology

To give you your hair the best chance to be in optimum health, it is essential that you are in a good state of mind. As touched upon in the chapter 3, psychological stress can lead to higher than normal hair fall which may or may not grow back and in some extreme cases, Alopecia Areata or patchy hair fall, which does not grow back. Psychological stress is not always easy to spot. A person can easily feel that he/she is in a good state of mind but they might be suffering from an underlying stress (e.g. chronic anxiety, depression or fear) that is so embedded into their day to day life that they do not even recognize it exists as a problem. Psychological stress has hamper normal bodily functions, disrupt the immune system, cause abnormality in hormone production (e.g. Cortisol) and cause inflammation, all of which have adverse effects on the health of hair and overall health. Having a positive, happy outlook on life in general and about health or hair specifically, can go a long way to tackle psychological stress. Psychological stress can be managed through professional counselling, positive image, having good people around to talk to and socialize with and so on.

It is essential to understand any psychological stress and tackle the root cause by whatever means, be it through a professional or taking specific actions to rectify the issues (e.g. make changes to working environment that might be causing grievances). Another well documented means of tackling psychological stress is through meditation. A form of relatively easy meditation is daily breathing exercises, which not only ensure adequate oxygen circulation throughout the body and head, it can also reduce psychological stress and help in relaxation. Visualization techniques (e.g. picturing a happy place) and positive thoughts are also good methods of calming the mind and reducing psychological stress. Also, having happy and optimistic thoughts and positive outlook on life generally, can go a long way in stress reduction. Finally, it is essential to not stress or worry about hair fall - doing this only increases the stress on the mind and can perpetuate further hair fall. Psychologically, the best thing to do for a hair loss sufferer is to not care about the hair fall (but carry on treating the hair loss using the methods described here) or to believe that the hair loss can be reversed (for example, through visualization), which will shut out any excess stress from hair fall and prepare the body to recover and re grow hair.

Physiology

Again, building on the concepts from previous chapters, good physiological state is essential for eliminating hair loss and being able to stimulate hair re growth. Hair follicles are just a very small part of your anatomy. You cannot just target the improvement of your hair follicles; your overall health must improve for the health of your hair follicles to improve. It is just like fat loss - there is no such thing as targeted fat loss (e.g. on your belly or thigh or face), you need to lose fat all over your body! Another thing you will need to appreciate is that hair is not a vital organ or tissue (although we put a huge vanity price on it that sometimes define our identity). Homo Sapiens are the only animal with hair (not fur) on their head. As hair is not necessary for survival, our bodies do not work very hard to preserve hair, as it would say, to preserve other vital organs like lungs or kidneys. In the hierarchy of needs of your body, your hair comes towards the bottom - your body will prioritize other things before it works to preserve your hair. So, your overall health needs to be in top form for your hair follicles to thrive, especially when you are susceptible to hair loss in the first place.

Hair re growth and hair loss elimination does not work in isolation. To tackle hair loss and to promote hair re growth, you must take a holistic approach towards the improvement of your overall health. Also, if you reduce inflammation throughout your body, it will improve the health of your scalp and hair. You will notice this theme throughout the book. There is a positive feedback loop between the health of your hair and your general psychological and physiological health - if you are in a good state of mind and if your bodily functions are working as they should, your hair is also likely to be in good health. You will also notice that taking good care of the health of your hair will result in positive side effects on other aspects of your health. For example, taking initiatives to improve hair health by, say, having Saw Palmetto supplement to tackle DHT naturally will result in the better prostrate health or having a good balanced diet with plenty of vitamins, minerals, proteins and healthy fats will result in healthier skin.

In a utopian world, you would completely avoid any internal and external toxicity or avoid exposing yourself to any harmful substances (which includes processed food, alcohol, un clean water, etc.). However, this is not possible. So, you should look to detoxify your body at every given chance. The best and perhaps the easiest method of detoxifying the body is through clean eating, drinking and supplementing (as discussed in chapter 3) as well as through good, positive lifestyle practices and choices such as regular exercises or intermittent fasting.

Environment

Homo Sapiens have existed for hundreds of thousands of years in a habitat that has only changed dramatically in last few decades due to the advents of industrialization and new technologies. Our body is not used to dealing with a lot of new elements in our current environment, neither is it used to dealing with artificial, processed food, ingredients and products. This is because our gradual biological evolution (which takes hundreds, sometimes thousands of years) has just not caught up with the way our environment is being changed (mostly by us humans). So naturally, our bodies do not respond very well to something it is not evolved to deal with - and our hair follicles are no exception.

Environment can play a factor in the health of hair as well. Access to clean water and clean air, avoidance of toxins and generally hygienic environment can help support the health of hair. A healthy environment is essential for preventing mental and physical stress and/or inflammation, which can trigger hair loss and adversely affect the health of the hair. In an ideal world, clean, fresh water from pure sources such as natural streams or mountains should be consumed and used for washing up. If this is not possible, bottled mineral water or soft, filtered water (with all residues such as limescale removed) should be used for drinking and applying to the skin or the scalp. Whenever possible, polluted air should be avoided and clean oxygen without any toxins (such as lead, pollutants and dust) should be inhaled. Breathing fresh oxygen is especially important when doing breathing exercises or meditating to reduce psychological stress and to help prevent physiological stress. A very good example of the environment playing a part in hair fall is when a patient is exposed to toxic radiation (intentionally of course) via chemotherapy to treat cancer. In general, any environmental toxins which are foreign to the body, should be avoided whenever possible and clean, natural environment or consumables should be sought out. These environmental toxins range from plastic residue that spills over to

Hair Transplant

An increasingly popular method of gaining hair back is through hair transplant surgeries. This process involves taking healthy hair follicles from the back or side of the scalp (areas of the scalp that has not balded) or facial hair or in some cases bodily hair, and painstakingly implanting individual hair follicles in the balded regions of the scalp one by one. This surgical process can take a very long time, can be painful and most certainly be very expensive. Whilst it is effective in gaining back hair relatively quickly, the traditional medications (such as Finasteride) prescribed with it, can have many adverse side effects. Even with these traditional non-natural medications, the transplanted hair can fall out if DHT compounds associated with Androgenic Alopecia or male pattern baldness is not treated, it can result in a relapse of hair fall again and will require hair transplantation surgery again. This cycle will require to continue, unless and until the underlying cause of hair loss is treated. However, if the methods described above are applied after hair transplantation, it will give the transplanted hair the best chance to remain healthy and not fall out.

Hair transplantation in scalp regions suffering from Alopecia Areata or patchy hair loss, are very unlikely to be effective. After transplantation, the follicles have a high probability of falling out again, as the white blood cells will (mistakenly) start attacking the hair strands. Again, if the underlying issue triggering the auto immune disease and the Alopecia Areata is left untreated, the Alopecia Areata will prevail, even with hair transplantation surgery.

Finally, you must persist and be extremely patient. Results come gradually with consistency and perseverance. It usually takes at least 40 to 60 days to see any noticeable change and the change will be minimal. However, over time, if persisted with, the methods outlined in this book will yield you the optimal results. To use an analogy, it is a bit like going to the gym or brushing your teeth - a few workout sessions or a few days of brushing will not give you any noticeable results, but if persisted with, you will see that you are getting fitter with each trip to the gym and your teeth will get healthier/whiter as you thoroughly brush your teeth day in, day out with a good toothpaste. Perhaps, the biggest gain is not the noticeable changes of persisting with the hair/lifestyle regimen suggested in this book or going to the gym or brushing your teeth; it is perhaps the avoidance of what would have happened if one does not persist - i.e. continuously receding hairline until none is left or obesity or unhealthy, painful, yellow teeth!

Other Hair Loss Factors

There are many other less common factors that may lead to hair loss in rare circumstances. Among these are hair loss due to injury or trauma, head lice, fungal infections, chemotherapy, etc. Again, as discussed throughout this book, the root cause of these problems will need to be tackled to eliminate the hair loss arising from these fewer common factors. For example, if the hair loss is due to injury to the head, then it is likely that the affected region has dead cells and is not getting blood circulation. The affected region must be stimulated to gain back the hair, but the effectiveness will depend on the severity of the injury (the worse the injury is, the harder it will be to re-vitalize). Hair loss due to head lice will need elimination of lice from the scalp through anti-lice chemical treatment. Chemotherapy patients usually tend to gain back their hair once treatment is stopped and the body is not exposed to harmful radiations.

New Innovations

Some new innovations in hair re growth is coming through.
Cyclosporine A, an immunosuppressive drug used to stop rejections
in organ transplants was also shown to have mitigated symptoms of
autoimmune diseases. While it was found to suppress hair loss,
Cyclosporine A had side-effects that made it unsuitable. Hence the
Osteoporosis drug WAY-316606 with similar attributes to
Cyclosporine A was tested to see if it stimulated hair re growth. It is
now in the early stages of clinical trial; however, side effects cannot
be ruled out and a date for the release of the drug as an alternative
to traditional prescription medication (such as Finasteride) for hair
loss has not been penciled in yet. Another exciting possibility of
reversing hair loss altogether comes from gene editing techniques
that are currently being developed. Clustered Regularly Interspaced
Short Palindromic Repeats or CRISPR is the cutting-edge gene
technology that could one day allow doctors or scientists to alter or
target specific parts of our DNA to eliminate hair loss (or change
any other cosmetic aspects of our appearance)! However, CRISPR is
at the very early stages of development. Aside from technical
challenges to safely develop a reliable gene editing technology, there
are many ethical quandaries that developers will need to grapple
with to get regulatory approvals for widespread use. Needless to say,
DNA altering could have profound side effects on our biology that
we cannot even begin to comprehend. For instance, if a person's
DNA sequence is altered to switch off the gene that results in hair

loss, it could kickstart hair re growth but could fatally enlarge the prostrate or adversely affect the immune system. Therefore, despite these progressions in science, as it currently stands, the most safe and effective way to eliminate hair loss and re grow hair is through natural methods discussed in this book.

General Principles

So, to summarize all of the discussions above about all the different factors involved in hair loss, how to prevent it and how to re grow lost hair, the key general principles must be adhered to for improving the health of hair:

I.   Hair follicles are just a very small part of your anatomy. You cannot just target the improvement of your hair follicles; your overall health must improve for the health of your hair follicles to improve.

II.   Listen to your body. Loss in hair follicle, especially when not gradual, is often triggered by underlying health problems or a change in your environment which your body is struggling to cope with.

III. Avoid anything that can might cause inflammation. Whenever possible, do whatever you can to reduce toxins and inflammation, be it through your diet, lifestyle or environment.

IV. Try to stick to natural, organic ingredients, food and products. Avoid unnatural chemical or medication that is not from a natural source and avoid toxic environments.

V.   To eliminate hair, fall and promote hair re growth, a lot of things, be it vitamins or hormones, must work together in unison. You will find that healthy hair maintenance will have a lot of positive side effects on your body - because everything in your body is linked, reinforcing point one above.

VI. Get as much diversity in your diet and haircare (more in-depth details in latter chapters) as possible to cover all bases, so that you are getting all essential nutrients internally and externally, for your hair follicles.

VII. Look to improve blood circulation to the head/scalp and feed it with adequate nutrients internally, as well as externally, using various and diverse sources/techniques.

VIII. Like finance, start investing in your hair early, when you are young, to get the best outcome. The less your hair loss is, the easier it is to reverse and manage and the better the outcome. If your hair loss is at a very advanced stage, where you only have a little bit of hair left at the back of your head, it will be much harder, if not impossible, to reverse. However, if your hair loss has only just started and you are young, you can easily control it and eventually completely eliminate it.

Conclusion

So, there you have it, a comprehensive guide to tackle hair loss from
all angles, strategies and techniques to re grow hair and maintain
the optimum health of hair. This method is 100% safe with no side
effects and all natural, which will not only improve the health of
your hair but will also improve your overall general health.

If I can help with anything at all, please do get in touch by emailing
me (navidayon@gmail.com) or through my website
(www.virileheath.com). You will also find additional tips, health supplements for your hair and hair products to stimulate hair re growth
in the site as well. You can also checkout my videos on my YouTube
Channel (VirileHealth). I hope you find this book useful. Thank you
for reading and I wish you (and your hair) the very best.

References

1. Tosti A, Camacho-Martinez F, Dawber R. Management of androgenetic alopecia. JEADV. 1999;12:205–14.

2. Hoffmann R. Male androgenetic alopecia. Clin Exp Dermatol. 2002;27:373–82.

3. Shapiro J, Wiseman M, Lui H. Practical management of hair loss. Canad Fam Phys. 2000;46:1469–77.

4. Gan DC, Sinclair RD. Prevalence of male and female pattern hair loss in Maryboroug. J Investig Dermatol Symp Proc. 2005;10:184–9.

5. Ellis JA, Stebbing M, Harrap SB. Genetic analysis of male pattern baldness and the 5alpha-reductase genes. J Invest Dermatol. 1998;110:849.

6. Nyholt DR, Gillespie NA, Heath AC, et al. Genetic basis of male pattern baldness. J Invest Dermatol. 2003;121:1561–4.

7. Sinclair RD, Dawber RP. Androgenetic alopecia in men and women. Clin Dermatol. 2001;19:167–78.

8. Russell DW, Wilson JD. Steroid 5alpha-reductase: two genes/two enzymes. Annu Rev Biochem. 1994;63:25–61.

9. Sawaya ME, Price VH. Different levels of 5alpha-reductase type I and II, aromatase, and androgen receptor in hair follicles of

woman and men with androgenetic alopecia. J Invest Dermatol. 1997;109:296.

10. Norwood OT. Male pattern baldness: classification and incidence. South Med J. 1975;68:1359–65.

11. Mulinari-Brenner F, Bergfeld WF. Hair loss: an overview. Dermatol Nurs. 2001;13:269–72.

12. Rushton DH. Nutritional factors and hair loss. Clin Exp Dermatol. 2002;27:396–404.

13. Sreekumar G, Pardinas J, Wong CQ, et al. Serum androgens and genetic linkage analysis in early onset androgenetic alopecia. J Invest Dermatol. 1999;113:277–9.

14. Vierhapper H, Nowotny P, Maier H, et al. Production rates of dihydrotestosterone in healthy men and women and in men with male pattern baldness: determination by stable isotope/dilutionand mass spektrometry. J Clin Endocrinol Metab. 2001;86:5762–4.

15. Kuster W, Happle R. The inheritance of common baldness: two B or not Two B? J Am Acad Dermatol. 1984;5:921–6.

16. Hayashi A, Mikami Y, et al 2015. Intestinal Dysbiosis and Biotin Deprivation Induce Alopecia through Overgrowth of Lactobacillus murinus in Mice..

17. Arck PC, Handjiski B, Peters EMJ, et al. Stress Inhibits Hair Growth in Mice by Induction of Premature Catagen Development and Deleterious Perifollicular Inflammatory Events via Neuropeptide Substance P-Dependent Pathways. The American Journal of Pathology. 2003;162(3):803-814.

www.ingramcontent.com/pod-product-compliance
Lightning Source LLC
Chambersburg PA
CBHW051401250726
48656CB00006B/2213